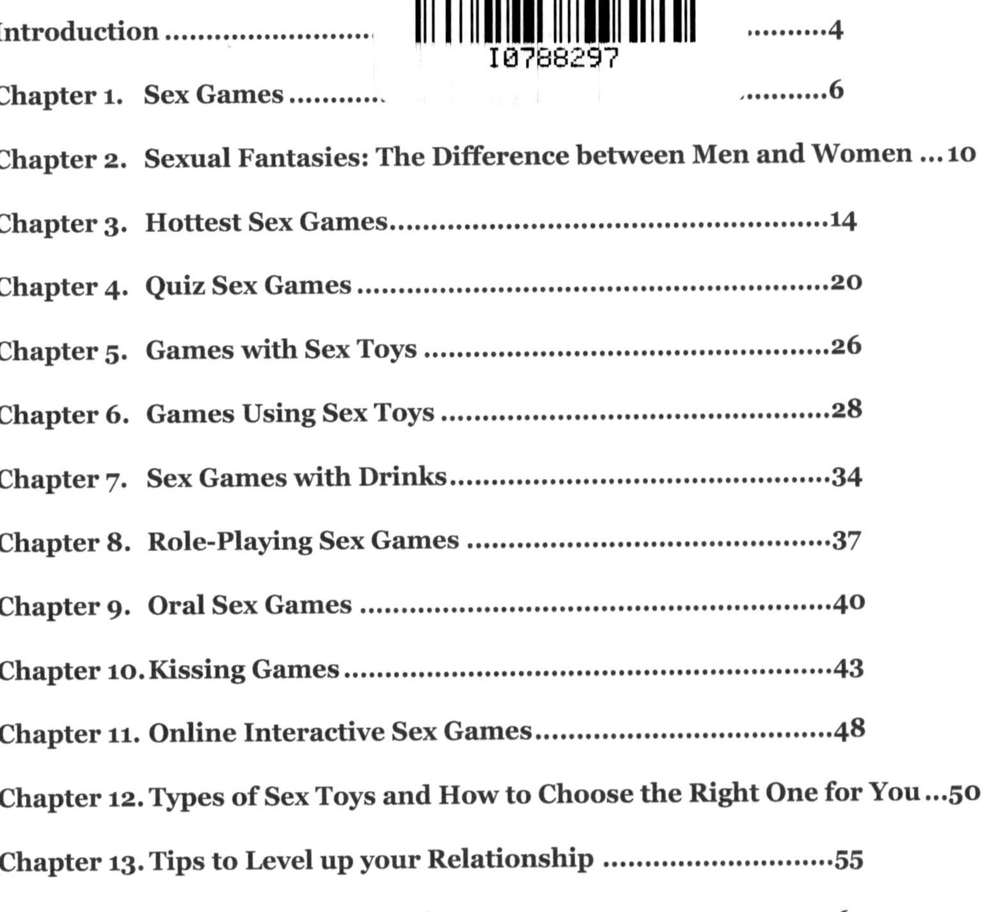
I0788297

Introduction

If you've been in a relationship that's like 99% of relationships, then your sex life is probably a bit less exciting and thrilling than it once was. In a word, it becomes routine, especially if you are living together with your lover.

In the beginning, you were in the honeymoon phase. That was when you couldn't get enough of them, and their mere smell was intoxicating for you. We ignore our other friends and obligations – even work – to spend time with this person, and sexual expression and release are a big part of that. This is a result of novelty and things being new between the two of you. It's a wonderful feeling that we love to bask in forever, but that is impossible for the majority of us.

If you're still in the honeymoon phase, then you may not need this book yet, because the slightest whiff of their aroma will be enough to make you quiver.

As you become more accustomed to someone, the honeymoon phase inevitably dies down because you start to see your lover as a person, and not just a concept of a being that you can have sex with. You see them as a three-dimensional person with flaws and faults and traits that may get on your nerves.

You have to succumb to other obligations and re-integrate yourself back into your life while balancing another priority: your partner. As if you didn't have enough responsibilities! There are so many people you need to catch up with! Your time spent with your lover might only be one or two date nights a week because that's all you have the energy for otherwise.

The point of this shows that despite our best efforts, our sex lives can grow stale quite easily. In some best-case scenarios, sex can be like a chore we endure at the end of the day when we just want to catch an extra fifteen minutes of sleep. In the worst-case scenarios, we live in dead bedroom situations – sexless relationships – with partners who function like roommates. None of this is good.

The bottom line is this: the partners have forgotten just how great and fun sex can be. That's why this is an entire book devoted to sex games to take your sex life to the next level or reinvigorates it completely. It can take you from strangers who pass each other in the night to that couple who can't keep their hands off each other. You will learn several aspects of sexual fantasies and how to introduce them to your partners effectively. There are many oral, kissing and role-playing games you will surely be excited to try with your man or woman. Different quizzes you can do to get to know better are included here too. Aside from that, all the things you are dying to know about sex toys will also be touched and which ones to choose and how to use them. As well as several ways to boost and enhance your sex life and intimacy aside from sex games are all given to you in this book. So without further ado, let's start learning!

Chapter 1.   Sex Games

Why They Are Important For Your Sexual Life

There are many benefits you can get when you introduce sex games to you and your partner, which are the following:

- Rediscovery

This is the first reason sex games are so beneficial for your sex life. Often when we drift from our partners sexually or have decreased interest in them sexually, it's because we feel a distance from them in general. In other words, it's not necessarily a sex problem; it's a relationship problem.

You may be well aware that sex is just one of the symptoms of an underlying cause. Regardless, sex games will help you tackle both the symptom and the underlying cause.

Sex games force you to laugh, work, and think together towards a common goal. It's this simple act of spending time engaging with someone in this way, and having fun that many people have forgotten. Imagine you are reading about one of the sex games from later in this book, and you are gasping from laughter while trying to figure out how to best adapt it to your situation. When's the last time you did that with your partner? That's the rediscovery of them as the fun-loving person you fell in love with, not the person who works too much and sometimes makes a mess in the bathroom sink. Having fun together leads to rediscovery, and sex games are nothing if not fun.

- Novelty

Of course, the novelty and allure of something new is also a major part of sex games. This is the feeling of first-time discovery rather than rediscovery.

Your sex life might be boring simply because it's boring. It might be too routine. You might want to try out kinks and fetishes that you saw in pornography. You might not even know what you like, so you want to try out as much as possible.

The pleasure of novelty in sex is well documented both scientifically and anecdotally. For example, are you more likely to be turned on when your partner has new sexy underwear, or when they whip out sexy underwear that you've seen dozens of times? That same lust for novelty is transferred over to the sex itself.

Sex games allow and push you to experience things you would never have thought of. If imagination isn't your strong suit, just leave that to me. I'll take care of that part and give you more than you can handle! You never know when you might see something that catches your eye and uncovers a trigger for your best orgasms. If you have the same type of sex with the same routines and the same lack of creativity over and over, it's easy to understand why your sex life is suffering. Try out some games and make it spicy and exciting again.

- Tension

What is tension in this context? Tension is the feeling of anticipation for something that motivates you toward it. Sexual tension is created when you have the desire, but can't necessarily take care of it at that moment.

Sexual tension is an important part of fulfilling sex life. Without it, you likely have no desire.

Sex games create sexual tension because that's how I've designed them! They are designed to open your mind and do something where sex might not even be the end goal. But, without your realization, you are more turned on and aroused by the game, until the sexual tension boils over and you just want to rip your partner's clothes off. Take the most obvious example of a sensual massage. Your partner orders you to strip naked for a full body massage and soaks your body in oil. They also strip naked. The point here isn't necessarily to have sex, but once the hands start gliding everywhere, it's probably where it will lead.

- Effort

Perhaps above all else, sex games represent intentional time and effort spent in the pursuit of better sex life. This is the most important part of fulfilling sex life – the notion that you must work at it, and it's not a given for compatible people. Many people assume that if their sex life with their partner is not naturally orgasmic, then it's a sign of the wrong partner.

How to Introduce Sex Games in Your Bedroom

You desire to venture the feeling of being excited about playing sexual games to flavor up your relationship. But there is only one problem. How do you convince your partner to participate in the idea of playing a couple of games with your partner? Will they agree to play this kind of game or be offended by the fact that you think your sex life is inadequate and boring? This is mostly true in long-term relationships; the idea of talking or modifying your sexual routine can also be inconvenient. But engaging in adult games can be a great way to bring new activities into your love life without feeling embarrassed.

Everyone wants fun and great sex life full of romantic intimacy, erotic adventures, new emotions and creative foreplay, and that makes them stronger. But most couples are not comfortable about telling the real deal of their sexual wants and needs. Most of the time, we just need a signal that it's okay to be alive, playful, and bad, to give us the approval to release controls over our sexual desire. The key is to start neutral by playing regular games first to build trust and confidence. Then increasingly switch to other levels of play, including more intimate desires.

This is a list of different varieties of adult-themed games with different levels of intensity. Try some games for each level or category before trying the next level. Adjust the speed you are going and be ready to level up if any of you stray too far from your comfort zone, sexually. Common games like cards, checkers, pool, and bowling let you play and have some good times together innocently. Try to make your partner comfortable with playing, and then crave the bet with a nice reward for the one who wins. Come up with a simple striptease if you seed that the mood is on and right.

Sexy games are made your emotional bond stronger by slowing it down and experiencing a connection with each other that is intimate. This can be real books or board games with questions and romantic activities. Also, a sensual massage or a shower gel for two can make feelings that are intense and erotic between you. These loving exercises will increase your confidence level so that you both feel secure with each other. Adult-themed erotic sex games can be fun, based on curiosity, or to wake up your mind. Obtaining more knowledge about sex and observing how your loved one deal with certain erotic issues can make you a more sensitive, sensible partner.

Camera games offer methods to blend different types of sensual pleasure. These playful foreplay acts let you playfully hold and postpone sex while you induce arousal and excite yourself in different ways. This will make one motivated to try with new sexual techniques and positions, which you may not be able to do if you are not part of the instructions of the game. Be more watchful of what you like and build your confidence in creative lovemaking expertise.

Roleplaying games are intermediate sexual games in which you explore secret desire and fantasies. You can unleash your inhibitions and let go of shyness by pretending and getting into different characters doing acts of erotic and sensual scenes. Maybe you can start by mimicking scenes from books and movies. Try them out using only your imagination before buying accessories and costumes.

Playing and having fun with each other is great for your relationship all the time. When sex games and having fun bring you great feeling pleasure and extraordinary sex, both of you are on the correct path. Building and gaining confidence can be started slowly, and you will see that your partner will greedily explore games and fantasies with you.

Chapter 2.   Sexual Fantasies: The Difference between Men and Women

Fantasies can be triggered by your imagination, or by external stimuli, such as an attractive stranger, an erotic picture, a book, or a movie. Whatever tips you off, as long as it's something that gets you off, it's fine to fantasize about it. Fantasies allow you to express your creativity in a sexual way. You may fantasize about things that you want to do but haven't done yet. You can fantasize about things that you did in the past that still turn you on. Or maybe there are some things that you know you'll never want to do, but they're still fun to think about. You can revisit your fantasies as often as you like.

You can feel truly liberated in your fantasies. Masturbation and fantasies often go hand in hand (so to speak), but fantasies also accompany sex for many people. If you are slow to orgasm with your partner, you can call on your favorite sexual fantasy to give your lovemaking a little kick. Fantasies help you focus on the erotic, thus making it easier to reach the point of no return.

If you daydream about how you want to make love, fantasies can give you good ideas, plus they can give you more confidence when you decide you're ready to put your ideas into action. Fantasies are also great for you if you think that you'd like to try a certain sex act, but you're not totally sure. You can experience it in your fantasies to find out if it turns you on before you ever consider acting it out. Sex therapists have discovered that fantasies can be good in helping couples or individual deal with certain sexual problems. If you put positive, sexually liberating thoughts in your mind, you may become less inhibited about sex. Through fantasy, you can confront your fears about sex and learn to enjoy your sexuality on your own so that you can enjoy it with someone else.

Top 10 Sexual Fantasies

1. Threesomes or Group Sex
2. Sex with a Famous Person
3. Sex with a Friend or Someone You Have a Crush On
4. Sex with a Stranger
5. Sex with Someone of the Same Gender
6. Force Fantasies, Being Tied Up, and Being Spanked
7. Sex While Someone Is Watching
8. Sex in Public
9. Sex in an Exotic Location

Sharing Your Fantasies

Before you get into deep with fantasies, let's discuss if it's okay to tell your partner your fantasies. You and your partner might decide to talk about your fantasies so you can both learn intimate things about the other. The more you share about your sexual fantasies, the more your partner gets to understand your thoughts on sex. Perhaps your partner never knew you had such a wild imagination, and he or she would love the chance to explore some of your fantasy scenes with you. These are positive reasons to talk about your fantasies. But before you do, you need to keep a few things in mind.

First of all, you should only tell you, partner, and your fantasies if you think he or she can handle hearing them. You must be positive that he or she already understands that sexual fantasies are normal, natural and won't hurt the relationship. If your partner has a conventional approach to sex, then telling your fantasies could be upsetting to him or her. If you think that your partner would freak out if he or she learned, for example, that once in a while you have same-sex fantasies, then there's no need to tell. It might be interesting to tell a fantasy like that one just so your partner can learn what your imagination holds, but it is never worth telling if you think your partner can't handle knowing. If you want to tell this person, then just be sure that you tell your fantasies carefully. What I mean is, tell your mild fantasies before you disclose your wild fantasies.

Second, if you tell your partner your fantasies, you might want to explain that they are things that you fantasize about while you are masturbating or just things that you daydream about, rather than what you think about while you are having sex with him or her. It is perfectly normal to occasionally think about other things or other people while you have sex with a partner. (That, in fact, even helps keep some people from cheating, because it gives them an outlet to pretend, they are with others.) Yet your partners could get jealous, or even feel threatened if he or she learns that you are fantasizing about someone else while the two of you are having sex.

One last thing and it's essential to remember before you start talking to your partner about your fantasies is to be certain that you tell your partner if your fantasy is things that you don't or do want to act and carry out. Convince your loved one that people do not always want to live out their fantasies! Ensure this is comprehended.

Let's say that you and your partner have talked about your fantasy of having a threesome—two and a man. You think you want to act it out, but you're wavering. You two have a lot of talking to do, and a lot of steps to follow before you decide if you want to go through with it.

If you're thinking about trying to act out any one of your fantasies, there are some things that you should do first:

1. Talk about the positive and negative consequences of your partner. (For example, a negative consequence of a threesome might be jealousy. A positive consequence could be that you have a liberating sexual experience.)

2. While you and your partner are having sex, say a few things out loud—almost as if you're acting out the fantasy—and see how it feels. (Keeping with the example of the threesome, pretend that there is a third person in the room, and role-plays the scene. Pretend you are talking to the imaginary third person.)

3. Get on and watch erotic or porn movies as a couple and look at the kind of sex you're interested in imitating. If what you see in the movie turns you both on, then you are that much closer to realizing that it might work for you. If the movie turns you off, it might not work for you in real life.

4. Talk out the details of what you expect to happen if you act out the fantasy. If both of you can come up with a script, you'll be aware of what will happen, which will make you much more comfortable, confident and safe of the whole scenario.

5. Ensure one another that when you're acting out these fantasies, you will not continue if one of you dislike what is happening.

6. Talk about it again to be sure you both really want to try it.

7. If you both feel ready, then give it a try when you have the time and opportunity. Good luck! Remember, if you act out a fantasy and you don't like it, you never have to do it again. If this is the case, you can still enjoy it as a fantasy—just stop trying to make it a reality.

But if you enjoyed acting out your fantasy, then you and your partner have added a new and thrilling aspect to your sex life. Some couples find that acting out their sexual fantasies is an integral part of their sex lives, and it gives them the extra excitement that they don't get every day.

Sex Games beyond the Bed

As you move from games to lovemaking, be creative — don't just opt for the same few positions in bed. If you've got some privacy, explore the rest of your house. The kitchen table is often the perfect height for intercourse. Try the counter for oral sex. Have the woman bend over the arm of the overstuffed chair in the living room for rear entry. The woman can also sit on the arm of the sofa and have her partner kneel on the cushions as he enters her. This is a good position in which to put one of your feet up on the back of the couch. Choose the side of the sofa that will best allow you freedom of movement and maximum G-spot access. The most important point here is that you should feel free to be creative and experiment. Take turns thinking up new places and ways to make love. You've got nothing to lose and a whole lot of fun to gain!

The ancient book of Kama Sutra tells us that good health (physical) and growth (psychological) can happen if we try to do something new out of our usual habits in making love. Always look into nature and find inspiration from it like how certain animals of the opposite sex are always sided by the side. Being out there in nature can give an element of erotic anticipation and mystery to our sex life. You will have more awareness about yourself and your partner when you get yourself to a place or scenario out of our natural environment.

Most of the time, it is hard in the current day to day environments, to get outside that will make you feel safe for doing sexual acts

If you have a backyard with ample privacy, you can modify the area ideal for lovemaking. You can also try doing at your balcony's swing, a sofa in different areas around your home. These things will surely add excitement and new feelings to your sexual life. Try to get inspired by how animals behave when having sex. Try to go to the zoo or watch videos online and see how animals go about it. Older adults believe that we can find animals as a source of inspiration in our own lovemaking. Use your nails to scratch lightly and your mouth to bite gently. Use sound to add to the variety. Groan, growl, whimper, howl, hum and moan!

Chapter 3.   Hottest Sex Games

The Bondage Game

What you need:

Get a set of handcuffs or rope, a blindfold, and leg restraints, if desired. Line up your favorite lubrication, sex toys, feathers, and other good devices for teasing. Set a sexy scene by building a fire in the fireplace and creating a luxurious and sensual spot for her to lie. Ask her to wear a sexy outfit of her choosing, or buy her a new outfit—every woman loves presents!

How to Play:

When she comes into the room, greet her with a deep, passionate kiss, and tell her how sexy she is. Serve her a drink, and then lead her over to the pleasure zone. Gently restrain her hands and tell her that her job is to lie back and enjoy the ride.

Once she's restrained, it's your turn to tease her as long as you like. Focus on her breasts and work slowly: Fondle and caress her breasts, squeeze and suck on her nipples. Next, move to her buttocks, then her thighs, and finally, her genitals. If you draw out the teasing sufficiently, she may climax as soon as you touch her clitoris!

To make it more erotic, restrain her legs, and add a blindfold. Use your favorite toys as you tease her mercilessly: Use nipple clamps. At the same time, you kiss her inner thighs, insert a vibrating butt plug as you explore her labia with your fingers, or use your tongue around and around her clitoris while you insert a dildo in her vagina. Stimulate each area, but then move away before she even comes close to climaxing.

Why is it Fun?

Send your lover a note or leave a sexy voice mail and tell her you to know she's been working hard and feeling underappreciated. You have a night of pleasure designed to help her unwind—and you'll do all the work! This is something that can bring a new sensation to each other and a way for you to show how good you are in making her reach orgasm!

Dominant or Submissive

What you need:

A pair of handcuffs, a spanking item, and sex toys if you like to include it

How to Play:

Let your partner know that you want to play robbers and cops together as a form of doing dominance and submission. One of you will play the one got caught shoplifting, and one will play the cop representing the law, as a cop or the dominant must be in control of the game. You caught here shoplifting, and now you need to arrest your partner. Have them stand in a corner, facing the wall with their arms and hands surrendering. Pat and frisk down their body, taking more time on their waist, bottom, genitals and breasts. After, handcuff your partner and let them turn around and command him/her to perform oral sex on you or else.

To make it hotter, you can begin with a little game of chasing your partner around the house and catch her then afterward tell them as a cop. You need to do a strip search and slowly remove their clothing while breathing heavily on their neck. Once you are done with your strip search and frisking, command your partner to get down on the ground, legs and arms on squats, face down. Search your partner on this position and fondle their vagina or penis until they are aroused, either they are wet or hard. Now's the perfect time to perform anal sex with a toy (if consent has been given)

Why is it Fun?

This sexy game of dominance and submission is a fun way to introduce you to this type of kink.

Drop the Dice

What you need:

At least 15 minutes of your time, sex toys and dice

How to Play:

Make two types of list and number them from 1 to 6. For the first list, distinguish six foreplay or sexual moves like kissing, rubbing massaging, biting, sucking and nibbling, and so much more. For the second list, distinguish six erogenous body parts or "areas like ear, navel, lips, areas below and above the waist, etc. Once ready, one of you will roll the first die and the other one to know the corresponding body part from the first list and what sexual action must be performed. Your loved one "wins" that sexual act or foreplay from you. Once they did what was asked, switch roles. It's your choice of how many rounds you want to perform.

Why is it Fun?

This is one hot way to do foreplay before the main event, and you can get creative as much as you like in making a list with your partner.

Classic Strip Poker

What you need:

Set up a sexy area in your house and a complete deck of playing cards. Try to understand ahead of time the mechanics of the game with your partner. For a classic poker game, every time you fail to win a hand, you have to strip off a piece of the clothes you are wearing. Set up a stash of coins and divide it equally for the two of you.

How to Play:

Start by Dealing out two cards that are facing down and one card facing up. Agree upon a bet (a dollar or fifty cents), then continue by dealing out 3 pieces cards facing up and the last card facing down. Highest to lowers Winning hands are the following

- The royal flush

- The straight flush

- The flush

- The full house

- three of a kind

- two pairs

- One pair.

The one who is victorious of each hand will tell the partner which piece of clothing he needs to remove. Look whether you can go and proceed to do this drawn-out fore playing until one is fully naked, then let the winner make a final decision on what sexual fantasy or act he wants the partner to do. Maybe you can also add erotic elements like using sex toys, or using only hand or lips and tongue to pleasure you.

Another version you can do to make things hotter is by letting the loser perform a type of service like massaging a part of their partner's body, sucking the head of the penis, fingering the pussy or licking the breast of the winner. Once someone is fully naked, proceed to a sexual fantasy game related to gambling like a gambler having huge amounts of debt to a loan shark and to repay, he or she must perform a sexual act.

Why is it Fun?

This is a great way to do foreplay and can have lots of variety on what type of punishment and rewards you can give to you and your partner. If you are the type who does not get jealous of seeing your lover do some intimate activities with other people, this can also be a fun and sexy game to play with your friends.

Timed Encounters

What you need:

A phone with a timer or a kitchen timer

How to Play:

Set the timer for a minimum of three minutes or even five minutes. Agree to use those minutes to perform any foreplay you want to do and stop the moment the alarm goes off.

Why is it Fun?

This creates instant arousal for the both of you that can finish off to great sex. Not only it excites both of you, but the feeling of being desired within those minutes will also make your libido higher.

Come and Follow the Leader

What you need:

None, just the two of you

How to Play:

Figure out who is the Follower and who's the Leader. The Leader follows their fingers and tongue everywhere throughout the Follower in the specific way that they desire to be touched or aroused. The Follower at that point needs to make similar moves and recreate them on the Leader. Switch roles the same number of times as you'd like.

Why is it Fun?

This is great in building up sexual tension and anticipation and is a great memory game that can be both fun and erotic for you. To make it hotter, use food like Choco sauce or whipped cream put on your body in patterns he must remember

Rip It Off

What you need:

Lightweight or old tank top, shirt, or underwear you don't mind parting with after the game.

How to Play:

Wear any of the items of clothing given above, and while on the verge of taking off clothes, tell your partner to start ripping off any of the pieces of clothing with either their teeth or hands.

Why is it Fun?

This a great prelude to rough sex, which is a hot way of making love. It fulfills your desire to be wild and barbaric.

Mirroring

What you need:

Props you like, maybe some sex toys

How to Play:

One partner repeats the actions of the other with maximum similarity. The game is simple but incredibly exciting. How to play: undress and sit opposite to each other, look into each other's eyes, trying to read thoughts and guess what your partner would like you to do with him. After a few minutes, share your observations with your partner, and let him say whether you guessed right or not. Maybe you will be pleasantly surprised by the wishes of your partner and look at him from a new side. In any case, such a sexual conversation is exclusively erotic and exciting. After it, you can make each other's wishes the reality.

Why is it Fun?

This is one way for you to show your partner how exactly you like to be treated in bed. It's also a great way for you to show them several moves you like to do to them.

The Full Course Meal

What you need:

Different Food and Drinks for each room in your house (you can also make the feel of the room more romantic by using dim lights or candles)

How to Play:

Cook or buy a five-course meal (cocktail or wine, appetizer then a vegetable dish or salad, a main dish and lastly a dessert), which must be placed in every chosen room in your home. Go to each room and eat what course is inside the room while doing an erotic move or foreplay move, and as you progress to other rooms, you must also amp up your move to a higher notch. Maybe start with kissing, to stripping each other's clothes, to sucking and some oral foreplay till you reach the main event.

Why is it Fun?

This is a fun activity that will not only make you enjoy food but a great way to build sexual anticipation and tension.

Back to the Beginning

What you need: Just the two of you

How to Play

A pretty simple game of trying to bring back or reenact the first you made love. Be detailed from where you had your date, to the place you had sex and try to reminisce how you first felt.

Why is it Fun?

It's always the honeymoon phase where libido is very high, and it's always good to remind both of you how it's like to be so in love with each other.

The Hiding Spot

What you need

Cloth to be used as a blindfold, a necktie or something to tie the hands and your choice of candies

How to Play

It's a game of hiding and seeks but on each other's body. Set who's going to be the Seeker and Hider. The Seeker will be blindfolded and his/her hands will be tied and will kneel on the bed while the Hider will get naked and will lay down, placing candies on several areas of their body. Once finished, the Seeker must now search the candies using only his mouth or by kissing

Chapter 4.   Quiz Sex Games

Sexy Questions to Get More Intimate

Asking questions to your partner can help you get to know them better in terms of their likes and dislikes. This can also be a good bonding for both of you, especially when you're on a long drive somewhere. Take turns in asking a question. Some of the questions you can ask are the following, but I know you can think of more, which depends on what you are curious to know about them.

1. What creatively sensual activities can you imagine doing to each other with?

- An artist brushes?

- A flower?

- A feather?

- Silk scarves?

2. If we were to make our erotic video for just the two of us, what would be the setting, theme or plot of the movie, and what kinds of sex play would we film?

3. What types of sexy clothing or lingerie get you aroused? What color and style of sexy underwear do you prefer, and why?

4. What is the "strangest" fantasy you enjoy and will admit to, but would never or could not do in real life?

5. Where do you most like to be kissed other than on the lips? What color lipstick do you think is most kissable? What color of lipstick do you think is the most erotic for oral sex?

6. If I was naked and pretended to be a statue standing perfectly still, what would you do with just your tongue to make me move?

7. If we were both sentenced to house arrest together for six months with no other responsibilities, what kinds of things do you think we would order online to make sure our sex play never got boring?

8. Have you ever fantasized about being a porn star? What porn star names would you create for each of us?

9. What types of sexy clothing or lingerie get you aroused? What color and style of sexy underwear do you prefer, and why?

10. How many different words, terms or names can you think of for?

- Female privates?

- Female breasts?

- Male privates?

- Buttocks?

- Anus?

- Anal Sex?

- Masturbation?

- Intercourse?

- Cunnilingus?

- Fellatio?

11. Have you ever had sex?

- Without any kissing?

- Without taking any clothing off?

- Before reaching the bedroom?

- Loudly so other people could hear?

- With other people watching?

12. While working out together at a gym, you discover we're all alone, and you're feeling naughty. Where would you rather have sex?

- On any convenient exercise equipment

- In the shower, sauna or tanning booth

13. What is the maximum number of times you can ejaculate in a day?

14. How do you feel about having sex while drunk?

15. What do you always want to do in bed and never do? And why have you never done it?

Would You Rather?

This is another question and answers quiz that both of you can alternately ask each other. Would you rather be one of the best ways to get to know your partner, especially when making decisions when given two different, opposite scenarios? You can see how similar and different the both of you are using this game. Below are some dirty would you rather question you can ask each other.

1. In a fantasy or role-playing scenario set in ancient times, would you rather be the:

- Priest or worshiper?

- Knight or the one rescued?

- Barbarian or missionary?

- Witch or inquisitor?

- Traveler or native?

2. Which would you rather have as a lunchtime quickie?

- Oral sex

- Intercourse

3. For mysterious reasons, you wake up with a mixture of gender traits. Which mixture would you rather have?

- Feminine features including breasts but with a penis and testicles

- Masculine features but with a vagina and clitoris

4. Would you rather be spanked or be the one to spank someone while having sex?

5. Would you rather not have an orgasm ever again or have an orgasm every hour?

6. Would you rather be blindfolded and not be able to see while having sex or not be able to use your hand to touch while having sex?

7. Would you rather have sex with someone with bad breath or have sex with someone who keeps burping?

8. Would you rather only be allowed to have sex in the missionary position or only be allowed to have sex in the doggy-style position?

9. Would you rather have sex in complete silence all the time or hear dirty talk all the way of making love?

10. Would you rather spit or swallow?

Truth or Dare

Here is a dirty version of the classic truth or dare you can try with your partner or even other couple friends (given you are comfortable to see them perform dirty deeds with other people) To start the game, the usual set-up is to have people in a circle with a bottle to spin on the middle and where the bottle's mouth point to will be a given a choice of truth or dare. If you're playing alone with your partner, you can do rock-paper-scissors. The loser will choose between a truth and a dare.

TRUTH

- Have you ever had a very inappropriate sexual fantasy about someone?

- Give all the surnames of the people you had sex with

- Do you prefer being submissive or dominant?

- What was the last porn you watched, and when?

- During masturbation, what's the weirdest thing you have done?

- If you can spend some money, do you prefer someone that talks dirty with you over the phone or someone you can have sex with physically?

- Have you ever tried threesome?

- Have you ever recorded your sexual activities?

- What do you think is the hilarious thing we did during sex?

- What did you think the first time you saw me naked?

- Tell me what it is like to have sex with me

- What do you want me to say while we are having sex?

- What is a sex position that you wish we would do more often?

- If we could make love in a public place without getting caught, where would you like it to happen?

- If we could go away on a romantic vacation, what is the 1 thing you would pack?

DARE

- Dare someone to undress you with one hand

- Dare your partner to try performing oral sex using one of your fingers

- Dare someone to close their eyes and let them guess what body are you using in touching them

- Dare your partner to pick a sex toy and use it for a minute

- Dare someone to be topless or bottomless for the rest of the game

- Dare someone to buy a sex toy online

- Dare someone to kiss your neck for 2 minutes

- Dare someone to arouse you without touching erogenous zones of your body

- Dare someone to use their teeth to get you naked

- Dare someone to give you a lap dance for 3 minutes

- Dare your partner to use their tongue to write a word that describes you on your back

- Dare your partner to take a video of him/her giving you oral fro 30 seconds

- Dare someone to kiss your stomach for 25 seconds

- Dare someone to give their best twerking moves for 20 seconds

- Dare your partner to sing a few lines from your favorite love song

Never Have I Ever

Some people call it 10 Fingers, and this game is a fun way to know dirty secrets and facts about your partner. To start this, both of you need to have your 10 fingers up and take turns asking never have I ever questions. If you are guilty of doing something, put a finger down. The one who will be the first to have all his fingers down will lose. It's up to the winner what he/she wants to do as a punishment. Below are some questions you can ask but I bet you can come up with more

Never Have I Ever.......

- had sex with the same sex

- tried using a sex toy

- had tried anal sex

- received a lap dance

- watched another couple have sex except for porn

- had sex in the pool

- paid someone for sex

- fallen asleep while having sex

- done a body shot

- gave a hickey to someone

- flirted with my workmate

- been to an adult store

- used a dating website to get hookups

- kissed and tell

- had a lover way older than me

Chapter 5.   Games with Sex Toys

As a carefree child, you loved playing with toys, especially bright and shiny ones, with all the bells and whistles. Why should that change now that you're a pleasure-seeking adult?! Bringing sex toys into your sex-play shows your lover your mischievous side, not to mention your spicy, try-anything attitude. Plus, sex toys have the power to intensify your sexual enjoyment and promote positive erotic pleasure for you and your lover.

Today, couples all over the world are trying to regain the love and affection lost in their relationship. Today's life is so stressed and complex that, without knowing it, we end up putting our sex life in the background. Sex ends up becoming a monotonous and routine activity and, before you know it, this lack of emotion causes irreparable damage. Thanks to the introduction of new and advanced sex toys on the market, many couples are rediscovering their sensual sides. If you choose to use sex toys with your partner, you will surely get more benefits than anyone can imagine. Contrary to popular belief, these toys are not just a means of entertainment in the bedroom. These simple devices can bring the couple closer together and help them bond like never before.

 Sex toys are now available in a wide range of materials, shapes, sizes, and purposes. The choice of these machines depends on the preferences and the level of comfort that the partners share. While you enjoy sex toys with your partner, you need to make your partner feel comfortable and relaxed. The process of introducing the toy into your room can be a little tricky, but once you start using it, the results are worth it. In general, the couple who suggest using these toys is the ones who initiate the process of making love with it.

The best part about using sex toys with someone special is that these toys release your partner's sexy sides, which you may never have seen before. The use of such toys encourages both parties to get rid of their inhibitions and enjoy the sexual session to the fullest. The improvement of the couple's physical intimacy is reflected in all other aspects of their life, making their relationship much stronger than before.

The concept of sex toys is not limited to vibrators. There are many other manuals and mechanical devices available that make the act of making love absolutely wonderful. Couples who are not in favor of using these devices on their body can also wear erotic lingerie and games, which are an equally effective way of enjoying sex toys with their partner. Variety is said to be the sweetener of life, and this claim also applies to the art of having sex. The more innovative you are in bed, the greater the closeness between you and your partner.

Ways to Introduce Your Partner to Sex Toys

Too often, even sexually forward women shy away from introducing sex toys into their relationships because they don't want their partners to assume they are not sexually satisfied.

However, some people who love sex understand the provocative power of sex toys. They know that bringing them into the bedroom doe snot express anything negative about the carnal abilities of you or your lover. On the contrary, sex toys can add new sensations to your sexual repertoire, enhance your sex life, and connect you more closely to your lover as you explore and experiment with new ways to share and enjoy pleasure.

Here are a few things to consider discussing before bringing in sex toys to play with under your sheets:

Let your lover know that your desire to use toys does not mean he is not an excellent lover. You each have individual wiring, and even Casanova might not be able to get you to hit that sweet high note. He actually can become an even more proficient lover by consenting to your vibrating desires.

Sex toys are not for your pleasure alone. Assure any toy-jealousy that may arise by educating him about the ways vibrators and dildos can also heighten his enjoyment. Also, emphasize that you can't do this alone—to get your rocks off, you need him just as much as your toys.

Reassure him that playing with sex toys does not make him gay or emasculate him if that is what he fears. Sex toys create erotic vibrations and motions, and the desire to experience these sensations is neither gay nor straight but is innately human.

Chapter 6.   Games Using Sex Toys

Hot and Dirty Scrabble

What You Need:

Get a Scrabble game and set it up on a cozy spot with several sex toys of your choice. Both of you must start to scrabble with clothes on. List and agree on what will be the sexual favor or reward of the winner.

How to Play

The goal of Hot and Dirty Scrabble is to form words that express desire, lust and love for your loved one. Try to think of words that can arouse and make them horny for lovemaking. Based on the words you formed, get each other stripping and performing foreplay activities. The one who can come up with the highest score of a word will be the winner and be the one to receive the reward you set earlier

Play the usual way you do with regular scrabble but with the following additional rules:

- For this version, terms that are slang are accepted as long as it is related to sex.

- If words are sexy and triggering, Multi-word combinations can be used (without spaces) (e.g., glass dildo, butt plug lick my)

- Only one piece of clothing per turn can be removed for stripping.

- double or triple time will be given for sexy words placed on bonus squares

Here are some words you can form to set off arousal.

- Shirt: I'll unbutton your shirt slowly.

- Flavor: Let me taste the flavor of this strawberry syrup when I lick and suck your breast

- Glass: Pleasure yourself with a glass dildo while I watch you.

- Black: Open your legs so I can please you with this black vibrator

- Paint: Use a clean brush to put lube around the clitoris and nipples

The Extension

What You Need:

For this game, an extender is used on the male partner. It is a shaft made to fit over his penis to create extra length and possibly girth. This can be done at home or perhaps a hotel

How to Play:

When the male partner uses this, he could be thought of as a new or different person to the female partner. Perhaps the two partners could simulate an affair, the female character is having. This could even lead to staying in a hotel room when the extension is used. It might be enjoyable to explore even the most normal sexual activities or positions with this extender, as the sensations could be completely new to both partners. Let the female player give the male a "hand job" or oral sex. The male partner may find new enjoyment in watching his big new friend penetrate the female partner.

Remote Control Orgasm Game

What you need:

Is a road trip on your agenda soon? Pack a new toy—a remote control vibrator. Pack some extra batteries as well

How to Play:

Before you leave for your trip, you surprise her with a beautifully wrapped package. She giggles and stuffs it into a bag and leaves it behind. You insist she put it on. The object of this game is to get her excited, and then bring her back down—until she is begging you to stop the car and do her—now! Tease her with it, arousing her, and then switching it off. When you get to your destination (or pull off the road into a rest area), give her an orgasm (or several) via cunnilingus.

• Start out by coordinating vibrating speed with traffic lights. When you get to a red light, give her a low buzz. On the green, accelerate.

• Or coordinate the buzz with music.

• When you come to a private rest stop, practice chivalry by opening her door, helping her out, and laying her on her back, feet up, on the front hood like a hood ornament. No privacy options? Lay her on the back seat.

• Keep the vibration on her clit for a few moments while you play in her vagina.

• Now turn off the vibe. Run a flat tongue up and down the inside of her inner lips.

• Turn your full attention to her clitoris. Tap the tip of your tongue up and down the sides. Swirl your tongue around it. Tap the tip of the clitoris.

• Suck and swirl her to orgasm.

Door-To-Door Vibrator Salesman

What you need:

You'll need a suit, briefcase, pamphlets, and, most important of all, a selection of vibrators.

How to play:

Just dress in a suit and pretend to be a door-to-door vibrator salesman. Try and surprise your lover when she thinks you're off at work or busy doing something else.

Ring the doorbell, then come into the house and explain that you have some very exciting products to show her. Take out the vibrators one by one, taking your time handling each one and explaining which are best suited for what types of play. Ask her if she'd like to borrow one and try it out (with you watching, of course)! Or for variety you can also try the one below.

Come into the house and lay down the rules: You can only show her the products if she's naked, so the first thing she has to do is strip down (or get into something comfortable, like a short and sexy bathrobe). What's more, you're going to demonstrate their effectiveness on her, whether she likes it or not. At this point, you can pull out some silk ties or handcuffs and bind her arms or legs to a chair leg. Then run through the product line one by one, taking as much time as you like to demonstrate just how effective the devices are for stimulation, teasing, and perhaps even orgasm. Ready to step it up a notch? Ask her swap roles and test the vibrators on you—maybe you'd like to try anal stimulation!

Good Vibrations

What you need:

Set a sexy scene for your night of pleasure: Build a fire, turn the lights down low, and put on some sensuous music. Have a blindfold ready and line up all your toys that vibrate, whether that's the cone, a miniature clit vibrator, or something in between.

Remember, this game is about using a variety of vibrators to tantalize every inch of your lover's body! Slowly undress your lover; kiss her deeply, and run your hands all over her body, telling her just how hot and sexy she is. Blindfold her and lead her to the vibrating pleasure zone. Start out slowly, perhaps using a vibrating wand on her neck and shoulders. Try a different vibrating device on various body parts: Massage her muscles with long smooth strokes, tickle her nipples with a vibrating finger device, and finally move to her genitals. Here you can use a vibrator to tease open her labia, switch gears to reach her G-spot, and then come back to her clitoris for the final climax!

To take it up a notch: Use a pair of vibrating nipple clips to keep her on her toes while you insert a vibrating butt plug or have her grind on a cone-like device. Once she's hot and wet, turn on that U-shaped vibrator and stimulate her G-spot and her clitoris at the same time. Let her ride the vibrations to heaven and back! Pick two or three of your favorite vibrating devices, and start at her toes. Moving very, very slowly, use each device on every inch of her, taking care to test every speed, pulsation, and pattern. Keep her guessing where you're going next and what it will feel like, and build the tension by avoiding the genitals until her clitoris is fully engorged!

Pleasure Party

What you need:

The Sexy Setup Invite your lover to a "pleasure party" designed for two. Tell him you have a special lineup of tools and tricks to bring him hours of delight. Set a sexy and sensuous setting: Build a nest of blankets and furs on the floor, light some candles, and put on your sexiest lingerie. Line up all your sex toys, but keep them hidden under a silky scarf.

How to Play:

Welcome your lover with a long and lingering kiss, then undress him partially and ask him to get comfortable. Tell him you're the mistress of pleasure, and you're going to demonstrate all the different tools. One by one, bring out your sex toys and use them on various parts of his body, building tension and heightening the excitement as you go. Use a vibrator to massage his neck and shoulders, and then buzz his nipples gently with a vibrating finger device. Move down his body and tickle his perineum or around his testicles with your device as you stroke his penis.

Use each device to turn him on for a bit, but don't bring him to orgasm—stop and introduce the next toy until he's ready to burst! Then help him climax in whatever way feels best!

To make things hotter, help your lover undress completely, and invite him into the pleasure nest. Show him all your toys, but then blindfold him and tie his hands above his head. Tell him he must guess the toy in question as you use it on his body. If he guesses correctly, you'll reward him with a kiss (or a sip of champagne, bite of chocolate, etc.), but if he guesses incorrectly, he might get a spanking or a gentle slap. Test your toys one by one and think creatively: Use your vibrating devices on different areas of his body, slip on a cock ring and ride him for a few minutes, then jump off and insert his penis into a sleeve. Keep him guessing until he can't hold back!

If you dare, try multiple toys at once: Insert a string of anal beads, and then press your bullet vibrator against the base of his penis while you suck him off. Pull out the beads just as he climaxes!

The Glory Hole

What you need:

A suction cup dildo, glory hole is defined as a small hole in a wall where the man will fit his penis in it, and the person on the other side will caress it. For this experiment, it would be good to find a dildo with a suction cup backing that will allow it to stick to a wall.

How to Play:

This may imitate the idea that another male person is remaining anonymous behind the wall and allow the two partners to play out different fantasies with the "third person." Both partners could take turns, giving the imaginary person "head." The female partner could use the dildo to penetrate herself while she gives oral sex to the male partner. In essence, she would have control over her penetration. The male partner could also use it for anal penetration if he felt so inclined. If an added level of danger is desired, the dildo could be taken places where a glory hole might be found, such as gas stations or public restrooms or adult theatres.

Chapter 7.   Sex Games with Drinks

It Takes Two to Tango

When we come to the point of talking about alcoholic drinks and sex games, one can't resist the opportunity to think about the different classic hot sex games you can do. To start, one just needs to have an empty bottle; it can be a bottle of your preferred alcohol. Simply turn the bottle around and act out the one being asked for. When the bottle points to your partner, different types of kiss must be given to you. Also, in the event that you need to add somewhat more flavor to the game, you can utilize whipped cream or chocolate spread which of course will depend on what flavor you preferred and if the end of the bottle points to your partner, he must lick it from your body and indulge in whatever food you chose to heighten up the sexual anticipation.

Sexy Coin Toss or Heads or Butts

The classic game of coin toss is transformed into a hot, sexy and dirty version that couples will love. At each flip of the coin, both of you must bet opposite, guessing if it will heads or butts. The one fails to think it correctly must drink one shot and take off one piece of clothing they have on. The games end when one of you is already fully naked, which will then pave the way to more hot and sexy foreplay.

Boozy Body Shots

One of the most classic and straightforward sexy booze games, all you need to have would be two pieces of dice, pen and paper, shot glasses and your favorite alcohol. Write on the part of the paper the different areas of the body and fold them, and indicate a number for each piece of paper. The player will then throw the dice and get the corresponding numbered paper. Whatever body part is written is where the shot of booze must be taken from.

Straight Face Is the Game

Provide both of you and your partner a piece of paper, each where you will list 6-12 naughty, dirty and erotic words you can think of without revealing them to one another. Once done, fold each cut piece of paper and toss them into a bowl.

With each turn, you and your partner will take one piece of paper and try to recite it so anyone can hear without showing even a bit of emotion. In the event that you and your partner can keep a straight face, no consequence will be served. Among the two of you, the one who will show a pinch of emotion, a grin, laugh or cringe must take one shot.

Hot Vodka Twister

Balance is the main concept of the game Twister, and adding the element of getting drunk will make it more exciting and way more fun. Play the game the usual way, but to make it different, put several vodka shots and some glasses with water on the sheet's number. After spinning, drink the shot on the number before you put your leg or hand on it. Lucky for you, if you drink a shot of water. All this drinking, touching and getting close to each other's body will inevitably end up in the bedroom afterward.

Steamy Eye Contact Game (Don't Blink Or Else)

Here's your chance to look into each other's eyes deeply without getting awkward. While looking into each other's eye, you must be still and prevent your eyes from blinking. The one who blinks will need to take a shot and strip off one piece of garment. This game will heighten the feeling of sexual anticipation and tension between the two of you. Maybe you can wear provocative clothes, so you'll make it more difficult for them to concentrate looking into your eyes.

Body Treasure Map (X Marks the Spot)

If you are looking for a chance and a reason to kiss your love, now is the best timing for that. In this game, your main goals are to remember where you want to be kissed and licked with their lips and tongue. Give your partner 4 chances in guessing where your preferred X spot is. If they are correct in guessing, then lucky for you because you'll be receiving some kissed and licking on that spot, but if they were not able to guess, they have to take 3 shots of your chosen alcohol. Keep playing, guessing and kissing all you want until the both of you are horny and drunk to finish it off in the bedroom.

Striptease Q&A

The first step in this game is for you to think of one word, may it be a thing, person, place, animal or emotion. Don't reveal the word to your partner yet. Give them 3 chances in guessing the word and let them ask you questions that you can answer with a yes and no for them to have clues. For each question they ask, they must give an answer, and if it wrong, your partner must take a shot and kiss you somewhere you like. If, in the end, they were not able to give the word, your partner must do lap dance and striptease for you, and of course, you know what comes next.

Blinded Erotic Touch

Blindfolds are known as one of the most erotic things you can use in doing foreplay and seduction. The reason behind this can be that when other senses are blocked, the remaining senses will be more sensitive. All feelings will be intensified, and a simple touch before will feel more intense when blindfolded. Having said this, if you want to make your next drinking session an erotic one, this game is something you must do. The first step is to have one of you blindfolded, then one who isn't will act as the guide and put the index finger on several areas of the body (better if its the erogenous zones) The once who has blindfold must then guess which body part are they touching. If your partner doesn't give the correct body part, he must take a shot, but if he does, you are the one who needs to take a shot.

Chapter 8.   Role-Playing Sex Games

1. In-Flight Rendezvous

What you need:

Make sure to set up the scenario in advance. Put on your sexy and skimpy flight attendant uniform, with high heels, lingerie and stockings. Put some props like what you usually see in an airplane like cups, napkins, snacks, drink tray and amenities given to passengers like eye cover, blanket and neck pillow. Of course, have your handcuffs ready to.

How to Play:

Tell your partner you planned an exciting game where he would act as a flight passenger, and you are the flight attendant who's going to give him lessons about the right conduct in an airplane.

As a flight attendant, tend to the passenger and ask him if he wants some drink or food, then make him do things that will annoy you like spilling drinks, asking too much and being demanding. Once you get too upset, have your partner kiss and touch you inappropriately. When you are fed up, say to him that you will be needing to restraint him, get your handcuffs out and put it on his hands placed behind his back. It's your turn now to take control of the game by doing what you like by tease or by showing your breast, touching his penis until it becomes hard. Make demands to him, and he must follow and make sure all are met, and you are satisfied. You can also punish him by removing his clothes waist down and arouse him using your lips, mouth and hands. Once you see that he's about to cum, stop to tease him more.

2. Act As Director And A Porn Star

What you Need:

Make a scenario of a photoshoot complete with a sofa with fur, or a bed with silk sheets or a rug in front of a fireplace. Set aside many sex toys and other props you can use. Let your partner wear her bikini or lingerie and wear a robe over it.

Put the film on your camera and additionally set up your camcorder or handheld camcorder. Dress up like it seems that this is true. If you really like your photographs to look valid, purchase a couple of pornography magazines and study the photographs.

How to Play:

This game is a great one for both of you as one gets to play an aspiring porn star or Playboy magazine model, and one gets to play as a director. Now, let's get the camera rolling! Instruct your partner that she must follow all your instructions since she's' new at this career.

Make your partner pose provocatively, sexy and sensual. Tell her to remove some of her clothes, play with herself, expose her bum, lean over suggestively and expose her lady parts by pulling her lingerie a little bit to the side. To make it wilder, have her wear handcuffs while you insert some sex toys in her vagina or anus (if she agrees). Get a shot for every pose she makes and compiles them to be watched by both of you afterward.

3. Serviced By A Housemaid

You need:

For the costume you will be wearing, you may opt to wear a loose housedress but with sexy lingerie underneath or wear a skimpy French maid uniform with gloves, white cap, apron and feather duster.

How to Play:

Tell you, partner, to get home early, and once he's home, encourage him to relax on a chair. This time make sure to tend to him like a maid does, giving him something to drink and eat. After this, you'll tell him that you have something that will energize him. Go into your room in a reserved and shy away and start cleaning up, but looking at him provocatively once in a while. From here, you can do a smalls striptease revealing your lingerie underneath, or if you're wearing the maid costume, you can remove it piece by piece and still treat him for a striptease show of his own.

Sit beside your guy and ask him if there is anything that is needing special attention— say you are at his service and will do anything he will ask for. Maybe he needs assistance in removing his clothes so you can put it in the laundry, or would he like you to turn on the television for him? Remove his clothing and leave the room. When you come back, tell him that should be you pleasing him and give him oral sex.

4. A Maiden And A Pirate

What you Need:

You will be needing a pirate costume for this one, whether by making one on your own or by purchasing one. Don't forget the smallest of details like the bandana wrapped on your head, darkened eyes with a patch, unbuttoned white polo, tights and pirate boots. If you want to go all-in, you can also use props like a pet parrot or hook for a hand

How to Play:

Inform your partner that you prepared a swashbuckling game for the two of you. You'll be playing as the pirate, and she will be a captive maiden. Make her dress up like one with a low cut dress full skirt with no undergarments and several pearl pieces of jewelry. Start the game by saying, "Ahoy, mates! Get your hands off the Captain's maiden!"Pretend to rescue her from other pirates, and you want her all to yourself. Pull her to your lap, stroke her hair and lay a kiss on her breast. Put your hands under the skirt and finger here and reach for the G-spot.

Another scenario can be: You're one horny pirate, and she's a captive. Tie both of her hands and do anything to here like sucking her breast, ripping her clothes off and licking parts of her body. For added pleasure, kiss her roughly while pulling her hair back.

5. Personal Sex Slave

What you Need:

Put on your best mistress outfit- a leather or latex bikini or lingerie, choker, decorative belt and armbands. For your partner, make him dress up with old ragged clothes, or he can be totally naked. Don't forget other props like a choker for him, handcuffs, and a blindfold.

How to Play:

If he likes being dominated, tell your partner you have something prepared for him. You'll both play the role of a mistress and a slave. As a slave, he must do whatever you will order him to do. Give orders like letting him feed you by hand, massaging your scalp or feet and let it progress to giving you pleasure. Order him to fondle your breast, suck on your nipples, adore your bum and tell him not to stop until you say so.

Afterward, switch roles and make him handcuff you. As his slave, he can order you anything he pleases like giving him oral sex or letting him enter you anally or just anything under the sun.

Chapter 9.   Oral Sex Games

1. The Sixty- Nine Ball Game

What you need:

Balls or a Pool Table

How to Play:

This is a sexy, dirty version of the game Nine Ball. For this version, a lot of sensual foreplay, stripping off clothes and oral sex will happen based on your skill or luck. So, the goal of the game is to be the first one to sink the #9 ball. In this game, it is okay if you do not sink the ball in orders, aka 1-9, just hit the target ball first. Anytime you are able to make both sinks and shot balls, you have the right to receive unique foreplay from your partner. The winner will be the one first to complete 6 games and oral and will win an erotic reward of full orgasm by oral sex.

2. Restaurant Server's Words

What you need: At least an hour, your usual date night outfit, sex toys you prefer.
How to Play:

The game will happen during a date night in a restaurant. You and your partner will be assigned lines or phrases and actions that you think your server will say or do during the meal. An example would be what a waiter would say when he's greeting you, bringing your drinks. While taking what meals you will order and when gives the bill. Actions and phrases will be given before you go to dinner, and all consequences from those actions will be fulfilled after the dinner, and you're home.

• "My name is ________, and I'll be serving you tonight = Blowjob for Him

• "For our special, I recommend the ______________dish= Finger with Licking.

• "Would you love some desserts to finish off your meal?= Combination of Oral sex and toy

3. Lucky Card

What you need: At least 30 minutes of your time, a deck of cards, sex toys
How to Play:

Each card deck number (1, 2, 3, 4..., Q, K, A etc.) is assigned a specific act connected to you and your partner.

Actions for each Deck, You may modify it too.

Ace – the man, will kiss the man on the lips for 20 seconds

2 – the woman will kiss the man on the lips for 20 seconds

3 – man will kiss and suck a part of the man's body

4 – the woman will kiss and suck a part of the man's body

5 – man will finger the girl

6 – the woman will give hand job

7 – man will lick the woman

8 – the woman will give blowjob

9 – man's genitals are massaged with a sex toy

10 – woman's genitals are massaged with a sex toy

Jackman is given oral pleasure

Queen – the woman, is given oral pleasure

King – 2 minutes of intercourse (everybody wins)

4. The Anatomy Test

What you need:

In a room, set up an intimate area for exploring such as a soft, furry rug or a bed with fresh sheets, you and your partner must undress and stay beside each other all naked, or you can also slowly undress each other, it's up to you. Review the different erogenous spots of the body and come up with funny names or codes that can help you remember it. Don't forget your necktie or handcuff, blindfold, and edible body paint.

How to Play:

Now that you are done reviewing the different hotspots of the body, it is time for the anatomy test! Put the blindfold on your partner and tell them to indicate the various erogenous zones of your body using one of their own body parts, particularly one choice among tongue, lips, fingers or hands. Once done, switch places, if using edible paint; put a mark on those hot spots with a ranking of how sensitive that zone is (1 for inner thigh, 2 for earlobe, 3 for nipples, etc.) Wear the blindfold and tell the numbers out where you want him to fondle using his finger, hand, lips or tongue.

5. Bring Out His Pleasure

What you need:

Set up an intimate, erotic scene like a bed with fresh sheets or a rug with pillows in front of a fireplace or candles surrounding it. Make the light a little dim, pop some bottle of wine, prepare toys and lube if you like

How to Play:

Call your partner and tell them you have prepared something specially made for him that he will surely love. What you want to achieve in this game is to delay his orgasm and prolong his emotional reactions or erotic sensations as much as you can. To heat things up, fondle his penis, lick the head, give him a blowjob or kiss and lick him all over. One explosive way to let him feel good is the ancient Chinese method called 3-finger draw. While giving him a blowjob, find the perineum, the area between the anus and testicles, then make a curve with your fingers and slightly apply pressure to it. This technique will make things hotter and harder for him.

Chapter 10. Kissing Games

1. Sexy Mood Match Game

What You Need:

With your partner, come up and list different sets of foreplay acts for every 13 values of the card from King to ace of a standard deck of cards.

Next is to Shuffle and deal out all the cards facing down so that you and your partner will have equal halves of the deck. Make sure no one peeks.

How to Play:

This game is a hot and sexy version of the Snap Card Game. This is a quick sex game where sensual foreplay, hot make-out session, and stripping can happen if you both have matching cards. Each type of card is representing an erotic foreplay act that both of you desire. Take turns in giving foreplay to each other to get both of you horny for the main event. Between the two of you, the one who gets to win more cards will receive an extra sexual reward or favor.-which will depend on what you wish to experience.

Both players will turn over their first card from the stack at the same time and put them facing up next to each other. Look if these two cards match. If it does not match, continue to flip over cards until cards match. At this point, both of you must shout the sexy mood is matching the cards. The on one shout first will win that foreplay. Instead of snap, shout the following words:

- If two cards are both red, shout "Lick."

- If two cards are both black, shout "Suck."

- If two cards are both red & black, shout "Fuck."

But in those instances where you shout the words at the same time, you must both perform the act to each other.

If you call out the cards wrong, you must face a punishment, which is the following.

You must strip off a piece of your clothes and surrender your cards to your partner if you called out the wrong type of matching cards. But no one among you will receive a sexual act or foreplay. If one of you is completely naked, you need to surrender your deck of cards.

If you did shout a match, but it does not exist, you must do the corresponding foreplay act as indicated by the top card of your partner. In this instance, you can keep your cards.

Shuffle and turn over cards facing down when one of you run out of cards then continue the game. You can play this on limited time of 10 to 20 minutes per set or per round or until will win most cards. The person with the most collected cards at the end of the game will win and will receive their special sexual favor or reward to be performed by the loser.

You and your partner can play as many rounds as you can, and I suggest you come up with a different set of foreplay acts per game.

Q-P	Hug and passionately kiss each other.
P-Q	Massage any part of your body.
Q-N	Tenderly stroke, caress and kiss an exposed erogenous zone.
N-Q	Kneeling, kiss and lick your belly, hips and thighs.
Q-B	Enjoy as you caress and fondle your partner's body.
B-Q	Expose and allow you to lick and suck their nipples.
Q-R	Sensual manual genital stimulation.
R-Q	Stimulate you with a sex toy (visual stimulation counts)
Q-Q	Ladies' choice of any foreplay activity for both of you.
Q-K	Orally pleasure you.
K-Q	Ass play - sensual spanking, massage, butt plug, etc.

Maybe you can also do another element of stripping clothes by making Jokers part of the deck cards. If both of you get matching jokers, the word to shout is "Strip." The one who says it last will need to remove his clothing using one hand.

2. Queens Gone Wild

What you need:

For a two-player game, prepare a regular chess board complete with its pieces. With your partner, make a list of different activities involving foreplay when a piece takes a queen or vice versa. Do write down erotic rewards for each piece that has the chance to take the King to finish the game

How to Play:

This erotic variation of chess is a foreplay game for your mind and body. In this couple's game, you'll focus on your queen. Play your queen right and your partner will do some stripping off clothes and pleasure you. Just like most women, in this game, your queen gets to play more than once. She won't stop until you're both have satisfaction

The main goal of the game is to let the King mate with the queen. You'll both have great rewards when you play with your queen a lot more because this is where foreplay happens. Make sure to take the queen to have more erotic activities.

Foreplay Activities Performed by Your Partner

Sex play Rewards

P-K	Genital massage to orgasm using lube.
B-K	Intercourse missionary style.
N-K	Intercourse doggie style.
R-K	Oral sex to orgasm while using a vibrator.
Q-K	Intercourse in any woman on top position.
K-K	Anal intercourse (winner's choice).

Make use of the standard rules of chess with a few modifications related to how the King and queen are played with. When you take a piece with your queen, your lover pleasures you according to the type of piece taken. And, when you get the queen.

- Strip of any garment you have on

- The queen will be placed anywhere on the half of your board by your partner.

- Your lover pleasures you depending on the way the queen was taken.

Primarily any activity involving your queen means your lover pleasures you in some way. The queen takes the queen's situation is exclusive. In this case, either choose one activity for both of you or take turns pleasuring each other.

You must move out of check unless you're in checkmate or stalemate, in which case you must still make a move with the King before he's taken. Once the King has been taken, the one winner will be receiving a special sexual reward based on the last piece of the game.

Play multiple games if you like to have foreplay of different intensities.

3. Bump and Grind

What you need:

For this game, you will need a Sorry! At the start, both of you must behave complete clothes on, ideally five layers and articles on to make the game longer and the sexual tension long. Afterward, sit together and make a list of sexual acts or foreplay acts for each card value, in this case, 11, and then mutually agree on the ultimate sexual reward of the victorious one.

How to Play:

This erotic and sexy version of the board game Sorry will have you, and you're loved on strip off clothes and act out several foreplay that will make your aroused and excited, to start the game, gather your pieces and put them around the board and home in able to win this and great sex waiting. When playing, every time you "bump "your partner, you bring them back to start, and you must say Sorry, but in this version, a little playful fondling will do the trick. Apart from that, you must let them take off a piece of their clothing whenever you send it back to start.

In playing this version, we will just some variation on the standard rules of the usual sorry game.

- Do the corresponding act of foreplay for your partner when you play a card, and you bumped your partner's piece.

- You must remove a piece of clothing to get ready for more fun to come in the event that you get to bring a piece of their home.

4. Crisscross Applesauce

What you need:

All you need is a fingernail, feather, or other small, gentle scratching device for creating the shivers. Set up a beautiful spot for exploration and keep some paper and a pen nearby for taking notes. Get naked together in whatever way you desire or come to the game undressed.

How to Play:

Remember the children's game Crisscross Applesauce? Then you know the goal of this game: to bring out the shivers on your lover's body. Have your lover lay flat on his stomach. Straddle his bottom, sitting on his rear end or lower back. Whisper this rhyme as you make the movements in parentheses:

Crisscross (draw an X on his back)

Applesauce (rub his back lightly in a circular motion with several fingernails)

Spiders crawling up your back (walk your fingernails up his back)

Spiders here (tickle gently under his left arm),

Spiders there (and under his right)

Spiders even in your hair (lightly tickle his neck, hairline, and head)

Cool breeze (blow softly at his neckline),

Tight squeeze (squeeze his neck or shoulders)

Now you've got the shivers! (Run your fingernails up and down his back or anywhere close by) As you draw the X on his back, gently sweep your clitoris and labia across his buttocks. Brush your breasts across his lower back as you walk your fingers up his back. As you blow softly on his neckline, run a finger down his spine, around his buttocks, and back up the crevice; alternatively, whisper "hot air" on his neckline and press your breasts into his back. For variation, use the Crisscross Applesauce game on your lover as he lies on his back and alters the words and movements to discover where he gets the most goose bumps sunny side up.

5. Guess the Flavor

What You Need: Candy with different Flavors like Jolly Ranchers or Skittles, Water

How to Play: Eat a piece of candy without letting your partner see the color or flavor of it. After eating it, let them kiss you and make them guess what flavor it is. Take turns. Whoever loses will give oral sex to the winner.

Chapter 11. Online Interactive Sex Games

Our technology today not only helps us simplify and make our lives convenient but also to make it exciting and fun. Games have been one aspect of technology that grew in terms of new graphic and animation features and pretty much attracted lots of people and players online. It's the same with how games involving sex has evolved. Going online, you'll see a lot of different online games of such nature.

In these themed online sex game platforms, usually, you control a computer-generated character that can be of a different race, look, and sexual orientation. Apart from that, there are available different levels of interaction with other users you should achieve.

Your characters online can be customized according to what appearance, dress and characteristics you like them to have. The player can also control the different activities it can participate in and what conversations the avatar can hold. For some, these sex games online can be a way for them to interact with real people, freely and with less hesitation. Interacting with real people can happen through chat, microphone or even webcams.

Though this can't be at par with real interaction, people use these platforms to meet new people they can hang out with or sometimes to compensate for temporary periods of loneliness. For some who are not that good with people face to face, this can be a way for them to boost their confidence and have that feeling of control. In the case of other people, using these online sex game platforms can be used to ignite and revive an active sex life. This is ideal for those couples who are in a long-distance relationship. Some popular online sex games are found on many websites such as porngames.com, interactivesex.com, playsexgames.com, and so much more. You can use any search engine you have and search for online sex games, and a lot of results will be yielded.

If you're not keen on using online sex game platforms, you can resort to some erotic apps to install on your smartphone. For example, there is Planet Pron, a wide selection of videos and free images to whet your imagination. At the same time, for couples' sex games, you can choose between Ultimate Sex Games for Couples for iPhone and The Foreplay Game for Android. If you want to try tantric sex instead, there is Tantric Sex Deck. The important thing is that the apps are helpful for experimenting. The phone must not become an annoying third party! Unless you decide to use it for sexting: if a couple is forced to stay away, they can still carve out a spicy moment. In fact, at a distance, you can exchange sexy images, perhaps through an app that does not leave a mark like Snapchat, and messages with high erotic content. The only precaution is always to be attentive to privacy, and to do sexting only with a person you trust, to avoid unpleasant inconveniences such as the diffusion of photos and screenshots of the chats.

Chapter 12. Types of Sex Toys and How to Choose the Right One for You

Vibrators

Vibrators can offer a world full of blissful orgasms. They not only help women discover what they need to blast off, but they also help condition our bodies for multiple or simultaneous orgasms. Plus, with their diverse shapes, sizes, colors, and functions, they are fun items to bring into the bedroom when you in an experimental mood. They offer a win-win solution to any relationship-rut problems!

- The Rabbit

This vibrator stimulates all the right spots, all at once. Insert the shaft into your vagina and press "play." The device will twirl and stimulate your G-spot, while the pearls at the base of the shaft stimulate the lower vagina. That cute little rabbit attached to the shaft packs a huge punch, too, stimulating your clit with its ears. Choose this vibrator when you're feeling experimental and want to achieve intense orgasms. In other words, this can be your everyday go-to vibrator!

- The Pocket Rocket

This is the most discreet of vibrators, looking more like a lipstick tube than a provocative plaything. Apply it directly to your vulva and your clit for some strategic sensual stimulation. You'll be amazed at the amount of zing this teeny-tiny item can generate. Being travel-sized, this vibrator is great for the on-the-go woman, and also is great for stimulating your lover's cock.

- Hitachi Magic Wand

This vibrator is great for massaging your lower back and shoulders—and some other delicious areas. However, it is more powerful than other vibrators mentioned here and can take some time to get used to. It has two speeds and a robust internal motor. If you find it too powerful, fold a washcloth in half and place it over your pubic bone before applying. The real secret to this toy's pleasure is keeping it in slow motion. Move this vibrator across your vulva more slowly than you would normally deem necessary. You want to ensure that every nerve is blasting off, and if you move too quickly, you may not get that effect.

- Talking-Head Vibrator

Need some extra-dirty talk when getting down and dirty? This vibrator is your ticket! Made of stunning blue or pink silicone, it has the same pearls at the end of the shaft and ears for clit stimulation that The Rabbit has, and it also has a voice-recorder computer chip that produces CD-quality sound. Record your own (or your lover's) dirty talk, or choose among prerecorded "fantasy chips"—French, Italian, or German lovers, or kinky dominatrix scenarios.

- The Strap-On Vibrator

Ever wanted to enjoy the sensations of a vibrator but still have both hands readily available to wander elsewhere? Well, want no more. The Strap-On Vibrator is a small vibrator that is held in place against your clit with pretty, perfect straps. While it is not as powerful as other vibrators, it is also not as intrusive a toy. Since it's on the smaller side, you can easily introduce it next time you're making love, and he can enjoy the mild vibrations as well.

- Finger Vibrators

This is a type of vibrator that is small in size and can fit easily on the fingertips. This can be used in foreplay and ideal when used in fingering and hitting the G-spot. Your partner can wear more than one finger vibrator, one vibrator inside your pussy and one vibrator on the clitoris. That would give the woman an intense orgasm.

Dildos

Dildos usually have the same phallic shapes as many vibrators but have no vibrating components. Many women prefer dildos to vibrators because they feel more like the real deal since they are made from lifelike materials like silicone and are the actual sizes of real cocks. Consequently, playing with one actually feels like having real sex. Plus, they come in all shapes, colors, and styles, so you can have fun shopping to find the one that is perfect for you! I suggest using dildos to not only stroke your vulva, labia, and clit as you would with a vibrator, but also for deeper penetration to achieve G-spot stimulation. You can go as gentle, rough, shallow, or deep as you like when indulging yourself with this titillating toy.

- Strap-On Dildos

While your lover has a phallic-shaped toy already attached to his delicious body, there are ways a strap-on dildo and a little bit of creativity can maximize your sexual chemistry! Remember, it pays to play well with others! Put a little spin on your traditional sexual roles, and have a naughty "what-was-that?!" experience. Playing with strap-on dildos is perfect for the man who loves anal penetration. He gets to experience the thrill of anal stimulation while you get to take full control of the thrusting and experience a rush of power and lust. Plus, a dildo will stimulate his prostate.

Having a strap-on attached also frees up your hands for other provocative pursuits, like reaching around and playing with his cock as you thrust into his back door.

- Double Ended Dildo

A type of dildo that has no base like any usual dildo would have, it will have two heads at both ends that are used by couples for double penetration at the same time. This dildo is mostly preferred by same-sex couples.

Harnesses

Go strap-on dildo shopping together at a local sex shop or online so you can decide which version of this sex toy will give both your libidos a real boost. Plus, viewing and reading about these toys can rev up your engines for some post-shopping nooky! Here are some booty-full basics about the equipment you'll need.

- Basic Harness:

This has adjustable straps that go around your waist and thighs with a spot to insert a dildo. Its simplicity makes it simply sexy!

- G-String Harness:

With a lovely leather thong attached to a slim waistband and a single strap running up the center of your butt and over your clit, this strap-on will give your over a large hard-on and give you great stimulation at the same time!

- The Jock Strap:

This dildo is attached to a waistband that has two straps passing around each thigh. It leaves your vagina exposed so your lover can reach his hands around his back to pleasure you as you give it to him, right!

- Vibrating Harness:

Oh my! This harness has two little vibrating pads attached, one next to your clit and one where the dildo comes out of the harness for extra anal stimulation. It offers intense his -and-her happiness!

Other Sex Toys

- Cock Rings

Cock Rings are one of the most infamous of male sex toys. Made of rubber, silicone, leather, or metal, they fit snugly around a man's cock and balls. When he's hard, the cock ring prolongs his erection by constricting blood flow to this area and keeping blood in the penis shaft. This means he'll last longer under the sheets, so you're able to blast off several times before he's ready to cum. Not only will you be fully sexually satisfied, but he'll also feel like a regular sex god!

- Nipple Clamps

We're not talking about the wooden clothespins of yore, and we mean the newly fashioned fun and stylish clamps that give nipple nerve-endings endless pleasure. For nipple-sensitive men and women, these items are a must-have! Choose the perfect ones for you.

- Tweezer Clamps

These are the best nipple clamps for novices. They are the most comfortable, and the tension can be adjusted simply by sliding the small ring closer or farther away from the nipple. Also, the narrow, curved, plastic-covered-wire ends close around the base of the nipple, so they leave a tip standing up at attention. This allows easy access for licking and teasing as your or your lover's nipples are squeezed in satisfaction!

- Clove Clamps

For the more advanced sex-toy player, these nipple clamps are big, sturdy, and slightly intimidating. The pressure is adjustable and is generally hard and rough. The gripper pads consist of mini-rubber disks with stimulating bumps, which also help keep the clamps firmly in place without abrading the skin. Also, there is a chain attached to this nipple toy. The dominant partner can tug on the chain to increase tension and enhance nipple pleasure. Oh, behave!

- Kitty Clamps

Again, this is not a beginner's toy. These alligator-type clamps have adjusting screws, limiting how tightly they can be fastened. But here's the kinky kicker—cylindrical weights are attached. Turn the dial and the clamps hum, gently stimulating the captive nipples. Up the dial, and the clamps purr with more passion and make nipples dance with delight!

- Butt Plugs

Butt plugs are designed to fit snugly and comfortably into your anus. They are typically cone-shaped, with a flared base that prevents them from slipping into your rectum. You can use them for butt play, to stimulate the endless nerve endings in your anus, or during vaginal sex, to give you the sensation of being filled by your lover, thus making the urge to orgasm that much stronger. An additional plus for him: the bulge in the middle of a butt plug stimulates his prostate.

- Anal Beads

Anal beads come in all different colors, sizes, and styles. Like pearls, they are knotted together into place along a string and have a ring at one end. You insert the beads into your or your lover's anus and one by one, pull the beads out. The sensations of the beads going in and coming out of your anus cause your sphincter muscles to contract, which feels incredible and can greatly intensify orgasms in both men and women.

- Vibrating Panties

This a type of sex toy that ladies can wear, underwear that has a vibrator attached to it that is controlled by a remote control where one can control the intensity of the vibration. This can be a fun playing activity for you and your partner.

Chapter 13. Tips to Level up your Relationship

Individuals who truly care for their partner want to extend the closeness and passion only lovemaking can bring. These people love to stay close to their partners (both physically and emotionally). After completing a whole round of lovemaking, many couples like to talk about things that are important to their relationship.

One of the most important parts of a great sexual relationship is the ability to share what you like and dislike about your lovemaking sessions. If you can freely communicate these things with your partner, you'll have great opportunities for improving your passionate encounters. That means you can enhance the overall experience brought about by the union of your bodies.

- Helping a Woman to Achieve Orgasm

If your lover hasn't reached a climax during sex, or if she likes to have another orgasm, but you are still not ready for a new round, you may stimulate her clit using your hands and fingers.

- How to Sustain the Harmony

In general, couples don't like to throw away the warmth of passionate lovemaking by simply falling asleep, or by doing things that are mentally or physically demanding. Some lovers want to lie on the bed and feel each other's presence, while others like to perform a gentle (but not sensual) massage.

If the couple wants to get up from the bed, they can sustain a romantic and harmonious mood by listening to music, eating together, or walking leisurely.

What You Can Do After

- After making love to each other, the couple should clean themselves separately. Once this is done, the couple must sit together–the man will apply some lotion to the woman's body.

- The man must embrace his partner and tell her how he appreciates her. Then, he should offer her some water to drink.

After all the hype and all the rules, it is great to sit back and enjoy the rollercoaster that life is. This will mean that all you will have to do is to love your spouse truthfully and while at it have serious fun. Staying happy in a marriage situation can be tricky, especially when the excitement dies down, and you don't have many secrets from your spouse. Below is a list of ideas that can make things spicier.

- Go on dates

Keeping the marriage flame after a grand wedding is often harder than many people imagine. Take, for instance, the fact that many couples fall out of love in the marriage years as a result of getting too used to each other. Well, one of the best ways of keeping the fire burning is to schedule dates. Every once in a while, it is great if both of you went out and engaged a date. This should happen randomly, but essentially, it should be a regular activity.

Going for dates brings many things into perspective. You will notice that your spouse is getting older, maybe they have wrinkles, or they are now afraid of drinking too much, etc. These small details are the things that help you stay together. Many couples remind each other of how premarital dates went, and how things were during the formative years. These things are the ones that often bring out the life in marriage.

- Have fun together

Many couples forget to have fun in the marriage itself. While they go out for proms, dates and adventures before getting into marriage, the wedding or arrival of kids is often seen as an excuse for a more 'serious' life. However, this should never be. A wedding is no license for boredom.

Couples must seek to go for that adrenaline-rich adventure together. Take a rollercoaster, drive across the nation, take random trains to nowhere, and go on cheap vacations and countless other things. The fact remains that you must make a deliberate effort to make your marriage funs and fulfilling.

- Listen to each other

It is a great thing to get married to your best friend and probably someone you have known for ages. While this may qualify as proof that couples know each other, it is never a solid excuse for ceasing to listen to each other. As you grow older, you must realize that each of you has picked up much fatigue, firstly from you and then from the world. This calls for more care, understanding and love as the years go by.

- Respect each other

Spouses need to respect each other irrespective of the years they have been in a marriage. As people grow older, there is often a mentality that things will change for the better by themselves. This allows the spouses to abdicate the duty of guarding each other's' hearts, being each other's' best friends and protectors.

Respect enhances relationships, even when emotions can no longer hold it together. The fact that a woman sacrificed so much for a man, or a man has gone through so much for the sake of the woman is often enough reason to earn respect. This is actually what helps couples married beyond a certain age. Many times, emotions such as love and infatuation are no longer common, and at this point, deliberate respect must be the glue.

- Improve over time

There is no such thing as a perfect marriage. A marriage must often be based on the ability of the couples to adapt to changes and development in each other, as well as in their environments to keep the marriage. This is precisely why people must be deliberate about improving the quality of a relationship over time.

As the years pass by, seek to understand more, to judge less, to be more trustworthy and many other things. Improvement can happen even to the most beautiful of relationships. The keyword here is to rely solely on your past only as a guide to how better the future can be. With such an attitude, you will rarely judge your spouse. Its hall always is a question of what you can do to cover for their weakness. This is the purest form of improvement.

Sex might mean different things to different people. Still, the bottom line is that it is a very healthy and natural activity that everyone enjoys and find meaningful even with all the different meaning by different people. Sex is not just about vaginal intercourse; sex can be anything that feels sexual, which could be vaginal sex, anal sex, hugging, kissing, oral sex or any sexual touching. Sexual activities are very important in a relationship whether one is straight, a lesbian, and bisexual, queer or gay or in any kind of sexual relationship. So basically, sex is any sexual activity that we engage in with our partners for sexual pleasure and gratification. We all know that there will come a time that it might become boring or like a routine if we do not spice things up, and this is where sex positions come into play.

Sex positions are the different sultry styles and ways of having orgasmic sex, and sex positions should be used just like outfits where different ones should be used at different times. Imagine having sex that makes it looks like you are in your honeymoon stage all the time. This is possible if you are acquainted with all the sex positions and their techniques. The fact is that with this, you wouldn't be able to keep your hands away from each other.

It is one thing to know about the different hot pleasurable sex positions and thrilling orgasmic styles that can be adopted in the bedroom. Still, the hardest part is being in the mood to explore and to try the suggestions and the new ideas out. The fact is that stepping up and trying something new might be terrifying, scary or uncomfortable for you, but there are a lot of ways you can help raise yourself to your sexual height to stop sex drought. If you always need loud moaning, the bed squeaking and having passionate sex with your partner, then you need to use and love different sex positions. Because it is only this way that you will be able to heighten the fire, the excitement, passion and mind-blowing orgasm that have diminished in your sex life. So, to rediscover your lost sexual desires and yearning for having sizzling sex. You can follow the under listed tricks and tips to get yourself to always be in the best mood for new steaming sexual positions.

- Get yourself a sexy masseur or masseuse

So, you can get yourself in the mood by first wearing kinky or sexy stuff to be more attractive, and then ask your partner to use hot oils to give you good soothing massages all over the body. This will help to reduce tension, and as tension reduces from all parts of your muscles, it will put you in a better mood to try your new sultry sex suggestions and positions.

- Keep installing the sex ideas in your mind

You will find yourself horny and needing good sex when you keep seeing an erotic sex picture in advance and how you will be having explosive sex under the sheet when you try out some very kinky sex positions. Make some noises, say sensual things and whisper sweet nothings in your partner ears ahead of time. Just go all naughty with your partner and talk dirty to prepare your mind for some very crazy sex positions that you will be expecting from your partner in the bedroom. All these will add up and make you want to try out hot sex positions and be in love with them.

- Spring up a surprise anywhere

There is something sensual and steamy about having surprise sex anywhere else in the house, especially in the shower, and a lot of couples like sexual encounters in the shower, so you can skip the boring bedroom routine for the time being and try other places and most importantly the shower. Surprise your partner, maybe in the shower with erotic kisses, demand some fingering from your partner and move your hands all over your partner's body and let your partners reciprocate the same till you get in the mood.

- Flirt and play around with your partner

You can get yourself in the mood for some kinky sex in advance by sending suggestive but subtle text messages to your partner to let him or her know what's on your mind. You can flirt with sending romantic and sex appeal messages to their phone; you can also sound naughty and dirty as possible to give them a clue about your moves.

Chapter 14. 5 Tips to Increase Intimacy

It is part of the reality that the connection between two people will decrease over the years, even though they began their relationship with a great level of passion and excellent sex life, though this can be a norm and, for some not considered a priority, a sexual spark in a relationship is truthfully an essential ingredient for a fulfilling and happy life with your chosen special someone.

If you observed and felt that the sexual spark both of you used to have is now fading, it may be giving you some anxious thoughts about what the future has in store for your relationship. Are you may be asking if that connection can still come back, and if it won't, what would happen to the relationship?

Several studies and cases with shreds of evidence on relationships and sex answers this question with a yes, that it is with a high possibility that you can come up with ways on how to rekindle and increase your connection with your partner, in all aspects including sex. For you to understand it better, we must familiarize ourselves with the best techniques you can utilize and how these can help you. Not only will these techniques help you revive physical intimacy with your partner but can also help in fostering a meaningful, healthy emotional and mental health.

To start, we will look at the different stages of intimacy so you'll be able to know where you stand and what you will go through as you address the issue.

The Stages of Intimacy

Being Infatuated: Basically, what people fondly call as the honeymoon phase where both of you are somewhat obsessed with each other. You are so elated and so in love and can't get enough of each other.

The Landing Stage: In this stage, you now see your loved one as a real human being who is imperfect and has flaws. It's one step down a pedestal, and adjustments on sharing life with them are being made.

Burying Stage: The stage where your energy is focused outside of your relationship (less time for your partner; rather, you are focused more on organizing, planning, fixing things for your gain

Rejuvenating: Now, you have a change of heart, and your focus comes back to the relationship, and you start to become aware of how attractive your loved one and all those flaws make him/her imperfectly perfect for you.

Love that lasts: This stage usually occurs in the fifth year of your relationship, and this is where the feeling of happiness, stability, support, love and security is felt by both parties.

Five Intimacy Techniques for Couples

Seeking the help of a counselor or sex therapist can be a good and positive step, you can take if you are struggling with your sex life. Through their expertise, it is good to help you remove your old, bad and unproductive methods of interacting.

For some who may find this step a little bit complicated and too tedious, you can do the following intimacy exercises to help you in increasing your physical, emotional and mental intimacy in your relationship. Go over them and apply all that seems helpful for you.

1. Respiratory Connection Exercise

Stressful and hectic schedule in life is the main reasons why intimacy in a relationship decline.

Knowing this, you must find ways on how to relax in order to increase your connection. You must encourage your partner to relax with you like listening to or watching about mindfulness is a great way to ignite something between the two of you.

Afterward, do this breathing exercise, which involves you sitting in front of your loved one and resting your forehead against them. Now, your eyes must be closed and take in deep breaths and slowly release it. With this, you'll find yourself getting more relaxed, free and lighter.

For both of you, doing this will give you the feeling of having more connection and good synchronicity because you are aligned physically, and both of you created a rhythm. This will then lead to a deeper connection like hugging and kissing, etc.

2. View of the soul

Both on emotional intimacy and sexual intimacy, the Soul Gaze exercise focuses surprisingly on the power to look into another person's eyes. Again, this technique helps slow your mind and focus your energy on your partner.

Experts recommend doing this at least a few times a week. It only takes a few minutes (maximum five), but it can have a profound impact on how you feel about each other.

To perform the Soul Gaze exercise, just sit in front of your partner and look him in the eye. Think of the adage that the eyes are a "window to the soul" and see what you are collecting from your lover.

What do you feel, remember, or desire? What do you think they are experiencing?

Don't worry if you're a little uncomfortable with this at first; Trust that it will be easier and more relaxing and intimate.

3. Give Tenderness for 15 Minutes

In reality, it will not happen overnight; you can't reproduce a sexual connection right away, yet you can methodically create habits and routines that amplify your odds of connecting with them at all levels. The method of the 15-minute sensitivity practice is that it will assist you with feeling increasingly comfortable being touched by your loved one. These encounters can get tense and on edge if your sex life is not that good.

Choose an area or space for the two of you then sit together, glancing in one direction. For instance, you can be close to one another, or you can stay behind your partner's seat. In this manner, a sort of delicate and fragile touch starts. It isn't unexpected to do this activity, concentrating on a brushing the couple's hair/kneading the scalp or even giving a massage.

You can explore different avenues regarding various methodologies and see which ones work best and satisfies you. Make these habits for the both of you or maybe even just for you when your partner is not available

4. Uninterrupted listening

You may not imagine that listening has a lot to do with the sexual connection with a partner.

In any case, when you don't feel explicitly close, it regularly has a great deal to do with feeling unvalued, and we feel that nobody is tuning in to us to listen. Once more, this technique or exercise will only be under 15 minutes for each individual. It can truly make you connected as one team again.

To begin with, set a clock for ten minutes. In this set minutes, let your partner voice out everything and anything he/she desires to tell you, maybe it be negative or positive. Listen cautiously, truly tolerating it, and don't make any interruption

After, when he/she is finished talking, think about what you have heard by repeating it and reflecting on your partner's primary concerns. You will be stunned at how significant and understanding it tends to be! At that point, reconfigure the clock and take the chance also to express yourself before your partner.

5. Sensuality and Consciousness

At the point when you wonder how to recover connection and intimacy in your marriage, you may accept that if it does not happen spontaneously, then it is not genuine. This tantric practice called Conscious sensuality can do something amazing for physical closeness and intimacy.

They start by taking five minutes to look at one another without flinching and inhaling deeply. At that point, go through five minutes stroking and touching your partner's torso, neck, and face before letting them do likewise with you for an additional five minutes.

Simply center around how it feels without essentially attempting to advance towards openly sexual actions. You can likewise try it if you like; however, you can likewise consent to limit this technique to kisses until you are not, at this point, agreeable.

Conclusion

Thank you for making it to the end. If I had to pick a few main points that I think you should take away from reading this book, they would be as follows:

Women and Men want you to take time and warm them up as much as possible. Do not rush sex and focus on how to build sexual tension and anticipation. Quickies are fine, but unless she is wet and ready, the experience will not be optimal.

Now and then, both men and women would love something spontaneous. Try new places and spots to have sex or perform oral sex to one another when your partner least expects it. Just don't get too boring with your routine.

Make sex a learning experience. Many couples feel that when they begin having sex, they enter a different realm. Do not allow yourself to get into this mindset. By making sex a different interaction, you make it more difficult to communicate normally. Don't be afraid to laugh and joke during sex from time to time and don't be afraid to try role-playing and sex games, and this will lighten the mood and make it easier to vocalize exactly what you want in bed. Make time during sex to have a quick discussion on what you both want, don't want and what you might like to try.

Watch each other masturbate. This can be an extremely helpful practice as it gives you visual information on what your partner truly likes. Sometimes it's difficult for a person to put into words how they want to be pleasured. By showing your partner what you like, you leave little room for misinterpretation.

Have a go at anything once as long as it's not harmful or harmful for both of you. Give assurance to your partner that they will not be judged for sharing their fantasies and desire to try something new or even considered taboo. Whether its willingness to try anal sex or have a prostate stimulation to having sex in front of other people, make your partner feel comfortable in suggesting new erotic ideas. You must respect your partner's likes and dislikes and keep a nonjudgmental, open, environment relationship all the time.

Sex is an important part of life and crucial for being in a fulfilling relationship. Whether you have a great sex life and just want to keep experimenting, or you're just starting to explore what makes you and your partner feel good, I hope this book has been a useful resource for you. Don't forget that this book is only a start. By opening up communication with your partner about sex, you can both continue to explore and grow sexually, figuring out how to have the most satisfying sexual relationship possible.

We hope you have enjoyed reading this and that it has given you food for thought on how you can add an element of fun and creativity to your bedroom (or other locations...)There is a limitless amount of other erotic roleplay ideas and games just waiting for you to discover them. Keep a journal of the themes and activities that excite you and your partner, and have fun creating your own fantasy experiences! Thank you!